I0441464

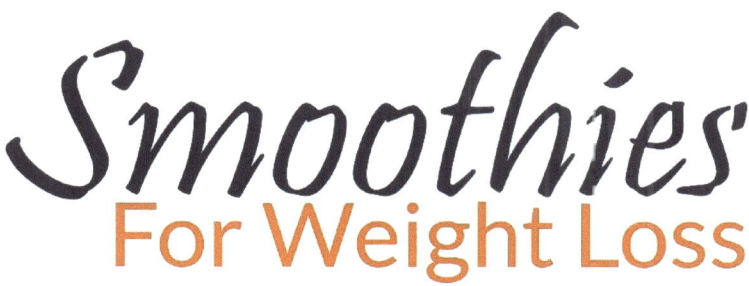

# Smoothies
## For Weight Loss

Copyright © 2016 Irene S. Marleene

# Table of Content

## Weight Loss Ingredients

## Recipes

# Weight Loss Ingredients

These are my favorite ingredients to use in almost any weight loss smoothie out there. The beauty of it is that you don't have to use each and every one of them. You can combine the ones that you already have at your disposal.

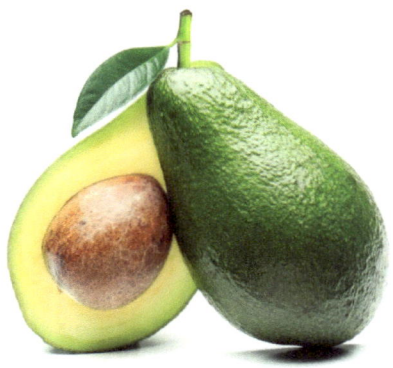

## *AVOCADO*

The creamy texture from the warmer climates of our world contains around twenty minerals and vitamins which makes it one of the most nutrient fruits out there. It is also known as the Alligator pear with monounsaturated acids making it healthy and delicious ingredient in any smoothie.

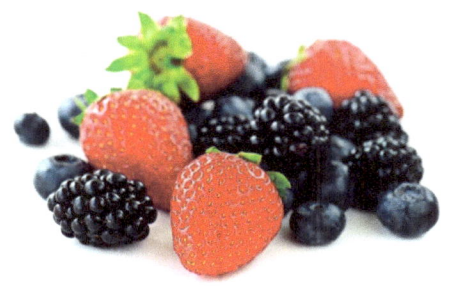

## *BERRIES*

All sorts of berries like blueberries, blackberries, raspberries and strawberries can give your smoothie some deliciousness and also increase the health factor because of their beneficial properties like low calories, f ber and antioxidants which can heal your body and help with body detoxification

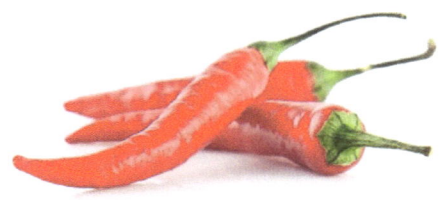

## *CAYENNE PEPPER*

The Cayenne Pepper is similar to the Jalapeno pepper, so adding a dash from this fiery ingredient in your smoothie can have anti cold, anti-headache and anti-allergies properties which also helps improving your digestive system and with that making it an amazing weight loss stimulant.

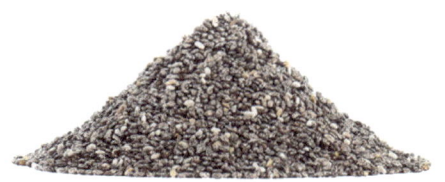

## CHIA SEEDS

Since almost all of the carbs in the Chia seeds are made of fiber making it a very low carb smoothie ingredient, it's very easy to choose the chia seeds as an ingredient to any weight loss smoothie. It will help you increase food absorption and burn more calories which is exactly what we are after for.

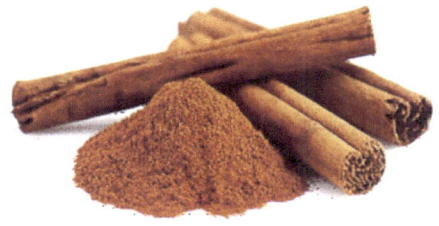

## CINNAMON

This ingredient can lower your blood sugar levels as well as prevent and reduce almost any heart related disease factor that you can think of. Cinnamon is one of the best remedies when it comes to stomach bugs because of the anti-bacterial preferences in it. The levels of anti-oxidants in cinnamon are off the charts and it means that cinnamon can repair damage to any part of your body if consumed once in a while.

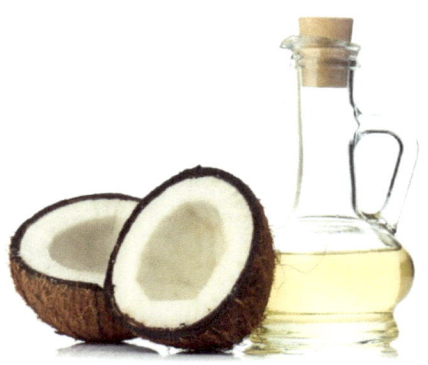

## *COCONUT OIL*

Perfect for losing fat, the Coconut oil is the ideal ingredient that goes well with any combination of fruits in a smoothie. This fatty acid is high in triglycerides that can keep your stomach satisfied until the next meal, without almost any fat whatsoever. The coconut oil fatty acids are metabolized completely different than any other low calories fat, that's why I use it in almost every fat loss smoothie that I make. Don't overuse it, just add one or half a tablespoon in your blender mixed with all the fruit to help you with digestion.

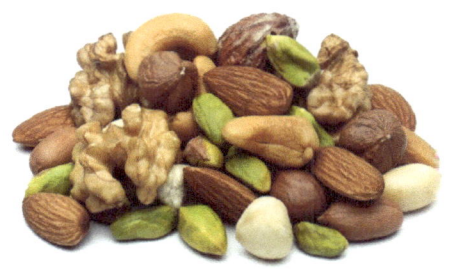

## *HEALTHY FATS*

Nuts, Olives, Soybean, Seeds, Canola, Walnuts are some of the healthiest fats that you can use when you are trying to shed some weight. The healthy fat contained in this list, have more satiety than carbs and regular fat making them the ideal ingredient in a smoothie that will keep you satisfied for a few hours without permanently storing the calories in your system.

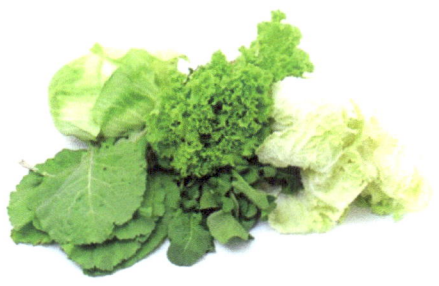

## *LEAFY GREENS*

Also a great weight loss ingredient that I like to use in my smoothies is any of these healthy leafy greens such as: Spinach, Cabbage, Lettuce, Kale, Broccoli, Collard, Dandelion and more. The nutritional benefits of these Leafy greens can help you lose weight while detoxifying your digestive system at the same time. Some of the nutrients contained in the leafy greens are magnesium calcium and vitamins such as C, A, K, B6 and much more, so do not hesitate to throw a leaf or two from any of these ingredients.

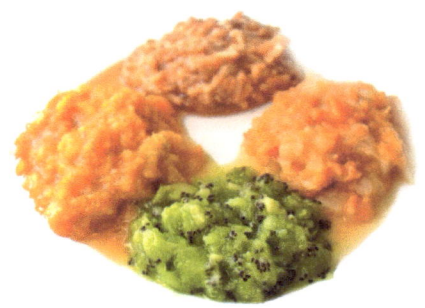

## *FRUIT PULP*

Instead of throwing out the rest pulp from your fruits, you should store them in a plastic bag in your refrigerator so you can use them as a smoothie ingredient later, because they are rich on fiber and you don't want to let them go to waste.

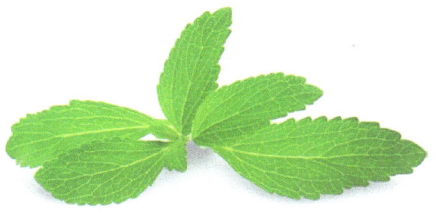

## *STEVIA*

Using Stevia as a sweetener instead of sugar for your smoothies is perfect because it will give you all the sweetness that you need but without the harmful properties of any other sweetener. Not only that Stevia will make your smoothie taste sweet, it's also not harmful to your health in fact it's very healthy because it has no calories whatsoever.

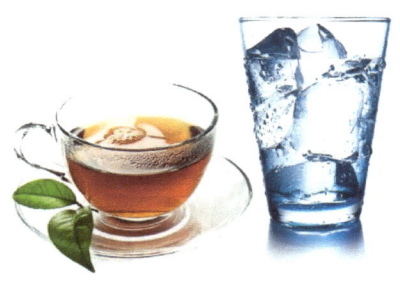

# *WATER ICE AND TEA*

Instead of adding milk as an ingredient to your smoothie, replacing it with ice, water or tea will do wonders for your body. It won't change the final taste outcome of the actual smoothie, but the difference it will make for your body is massive, so don't hesitate to use either of these three ingredients in any smoothie that you make.

# Blueberry Shock

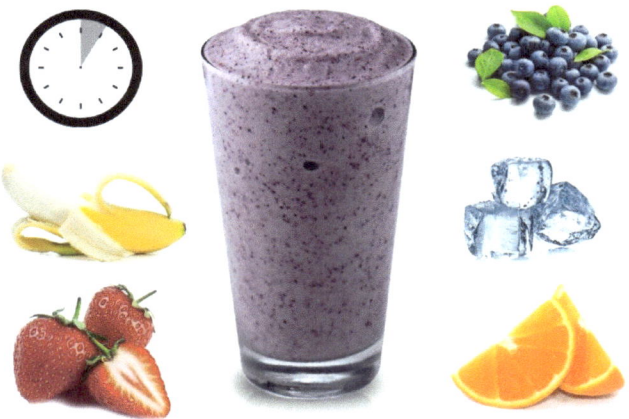

One of my personal favorite breakfast smoothies, a really great way to start your day. Very low on calories, this smoothie can be prepared in about five minutes and it tastes delicious. The level of anti-oxidants in this particular smoothie are very high so it will aid in weight loss significantly.

*Blueberry **Shock Ingredients:***

- *½ of a Banana*
- *½ cup of frozen Blueberries*
- *1 teaspoon of Coconut oil*
- *½ teaspoon of Chia Seeds*
- *8 ounces (230 ml) of Water*
- *½ tablespoon of Honey*
- *1/3 cup of soy milk*
- *Squeeze 2 small pieces of Orange*
- *½ cup of ice cubes*

Add all of the ingredients in your blender, Break the Banana in several pieces and blend until chunked or smooth depends on which of those two you prefer the most. Pour into one tall glass and Enjoy.

# Kiwi - Dewie

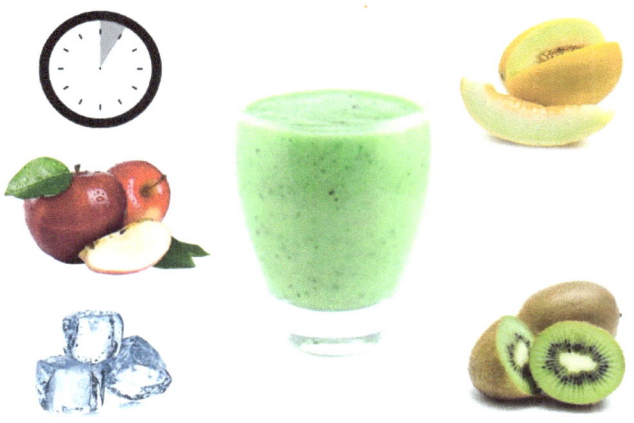

Rich on Vitamin C, This Smoothie will not only boost your weight loss, it will give your immune system the necessary protection from cardiovascular diseases and it will prevent your skin from wrinkling.

### *Kiwi Dewie Ingredients:*
- *1 Kiwi Chopped and peeled*
- *½ cup of ice cubes*

- *1 apple*
- *Dissolve one teaspoon of Stevia*
- *2 cups of cubed Honeydew*
- *1 tablespoon of lemon juice*

Place the Kiwi, Honeydew cubes and the Apple into the blender and Blend for 3 seconds. Open the lid from the blender and add the Ice cubes, Stevia, and Lemon juice. Close the lid and proceed with blending the ingredients until you think it gets the perfect smoothie texture for you. Enjoy

# Orange Sunrise

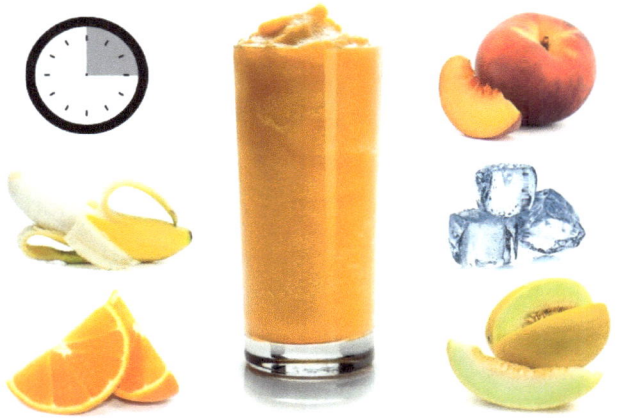

One of the best ways to wake up in the morning is with a fresh Orange Sunrise Smoothie to lubricate your entire body. Rich on Calcium, Fiber and acids.

*Orange* **Sunrise Ingredients:**

- *1 Banana Frozen and sliced*
- *1 Peach Sliced and peeled*
- *½ a cup Honeydew melon sliced on cubes*
- *½ cup ice*
- *2 teaspoons low fat orange yogurt*
- *½ teaspoon Stevia "sugar"*
- *½ Orange peeled*

Combine all of these ingredients in the blender and blend until chunked or smooth depends on which of those two you prefer the most. Pour into one tall glass and Enjoy.

# Tropical Mist

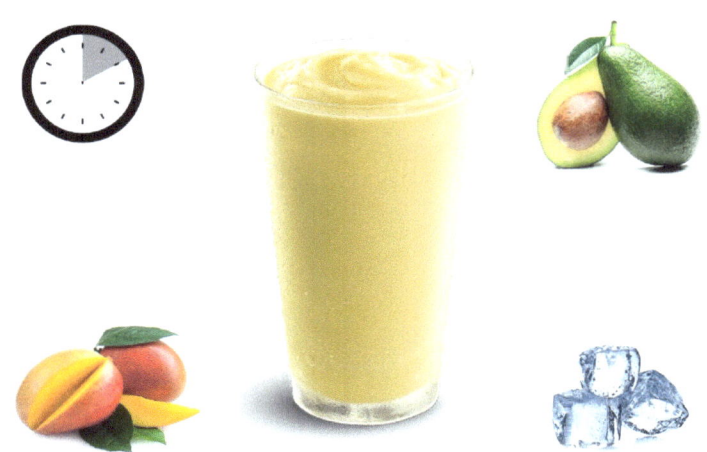

Keep in mind that Avocados have the good fat, but don't use too much, just a quarter of a cup filled with mashed Avocado should be just enough to add the wanted delicious texture to the smoothie.

### *Tropical* Mist Ingredients:
- **¼ cup of mashed ripe Avocado**

- *¼ cup of cubed Mango*
- *¼ cup of low fat (or 0% fat) Vanilla yogurt*
- *1 tablespoon of Stevia sugar*
- *5 ice cubes*
- *1 table spoon of coconut oil*

Add all the ingredients and blend them together until you see the desired texture of your choice. Enjoy

# Peach Delight

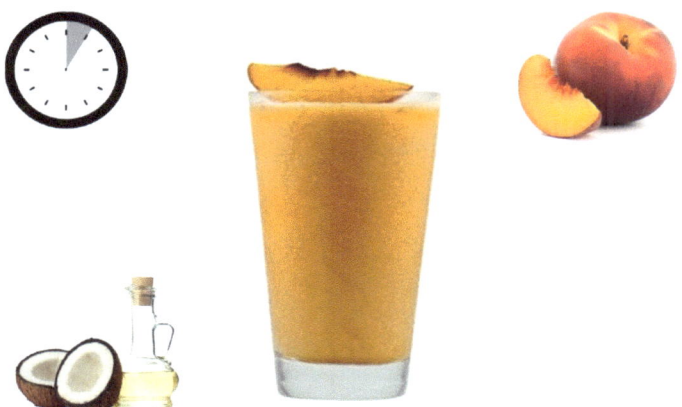

This is one of the easiest smoothies to make because it takes almost no time to prepare and it has only few ingredients, making it the perfect smoothie when you're in a hurry.

### *Peach Delight Ingredients:*
- *1 cup of frozen Peaches*

- *1 cup of soy/skim milk*
- *1 tablespoon of coconut/flaxseed oil*

Blend the peaches and milk for 5 seconds, open the lid of the blender and add 1 spoon of coconut/flaxseed oil and continue to blend until you reach the suitable texture of the smoothie.

# Peanut Banana

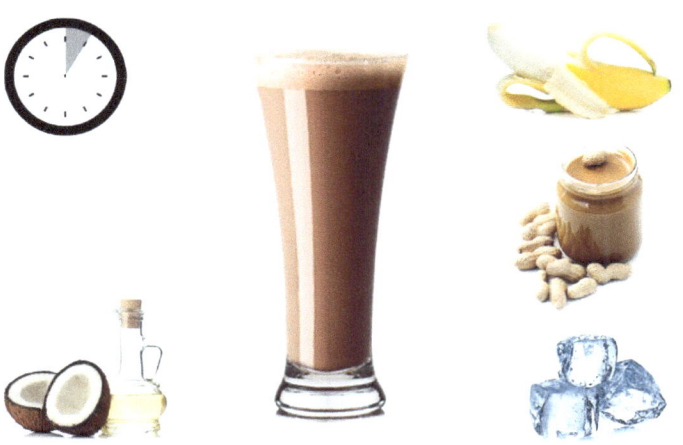

Don't let the word Peanut Butter scare you when it comes to weight loss smoothies, actually the proteins in the peanut butter are more useful than harmful when you are trying to shed some pounds/kilograms. Just make sure that you use the right low fat peanut butter and you can lose some weight while you still enjoy some sweet smoothies.

*Peanut Banana Recipe:*

- *½ cup of crunchy or smooth plow-fat Peanut butter*
- *½ of a Banana*
- *5 ice cubes*
- *½ cup of non-fat Milk*
- *½ tablespoon of Chia seeds*

Blend all the ingredients at once until the desired texture.

# Bloody Watermelon

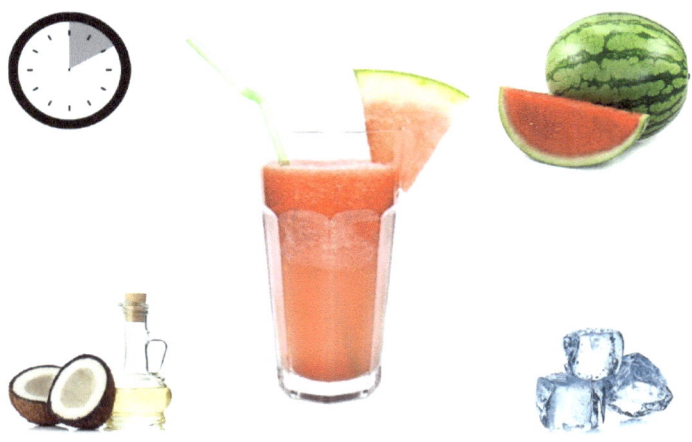

One of the most refreshing summer smoothies is the Bloody Watermelon Delicacy. This smoothie is rich on vitamins C, A, B6, B1, potassium, magnesium, and contains loads of fiber which is perfect for some weight loss.

### *Bloody* Watermelon Recipe:

- *5 cups of chopped and seedless Watermelon*
- *1 cup of non-fat milk*
- *½ tablespoon of Cinnamon*
- *10 ice cubes*

Put half of the watermelon in the blender and blend for 10 seconds, open the lid and add the rest of the watermelon and all of the other ingredients. Blend until smooth.

# Berry Remix

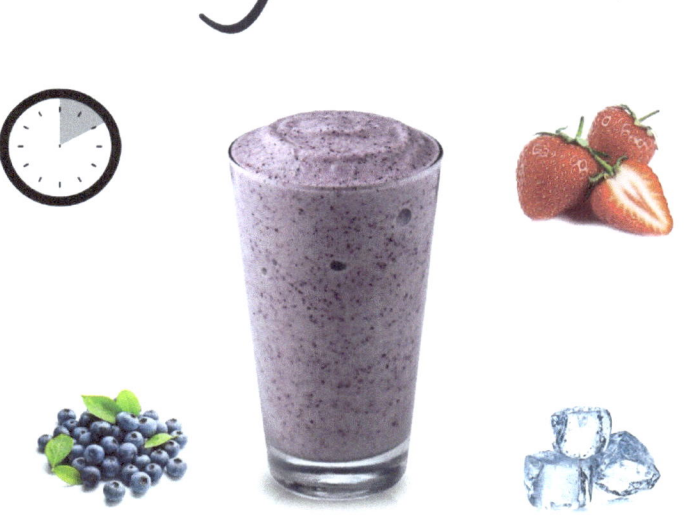

This delicious mix of ingredients can be made all year round. You can keep any type of berries in the freezer and they will still have the freshness that your smoothie needs.

### *Berry Remix Recipe:*

- ***1 and a half cup of frozen berries***

- *5 cubes of ice*
- *½ cup of non-fat fruit yogurt of your choice*

Blend all of the ingredients at the same time until smooth or crunchy, depends on your personal preference of taste. Enjoy

# 9

# Lemon Drops

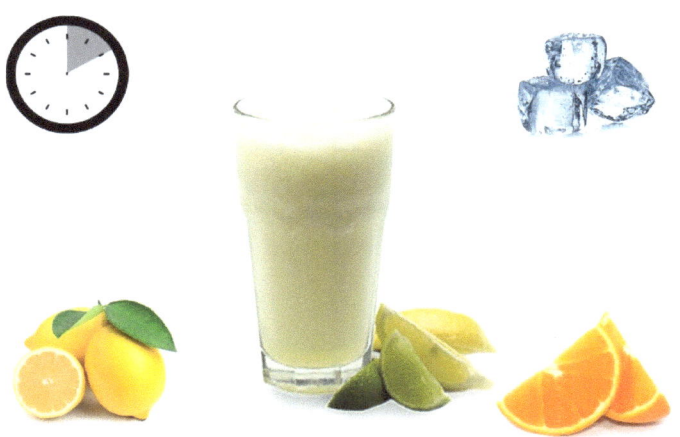

This combination of fruits contains the maximum amount of fat burning acids, and enough anti-oxidants for an entire day.

### Lemon Drops Recipe:
- **4 tablespoons of low fat Lemon yogurt**

- *1 tablespoon of Fruit pulp left overs*
- *1 peeled Orange*
- *5 ice cubes*
- *1 cup of soy Milk*

Blend the Orange, Lemon Yogurt, and the Ice for about 30 seconds before adding the Fruit pulp and soy Milk, again finish blending when you think it's enough for you.

# 10

# Apple Heaven

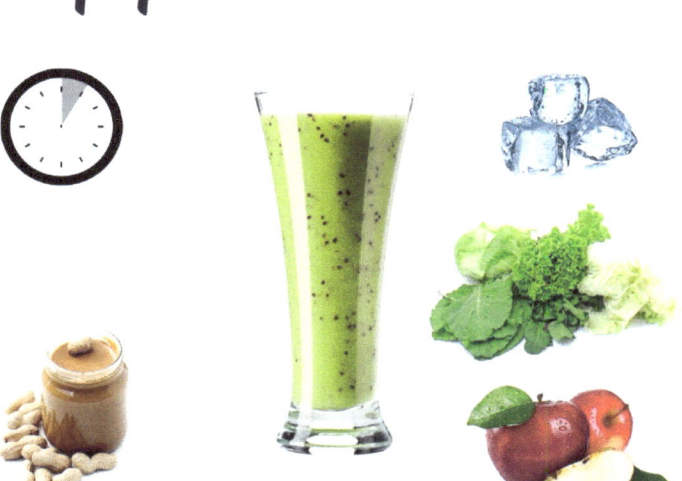

Apples contain a massive amount of Cardiovascular (heart) benefits, and that's why I love having this rich on fiber nutrient Smoothie almost every night instead of dinner.

### Apple Heaven
- **1 sliced Apple**

- *½ tablespoon of low-fat Peanut butter*
- *7 ice cubes*
- *4 tablespoons of low-fat Vanilla yogurt*
- *1 teaspoon of Stevia sugar*
- *1 Lettuce Leaf for extra nutrition*
- *½ tablespoon of Chia Seeds*

Blend until chunky because I prefer to eat this smoothie with a spoon.

# 11

# Mocha Delish

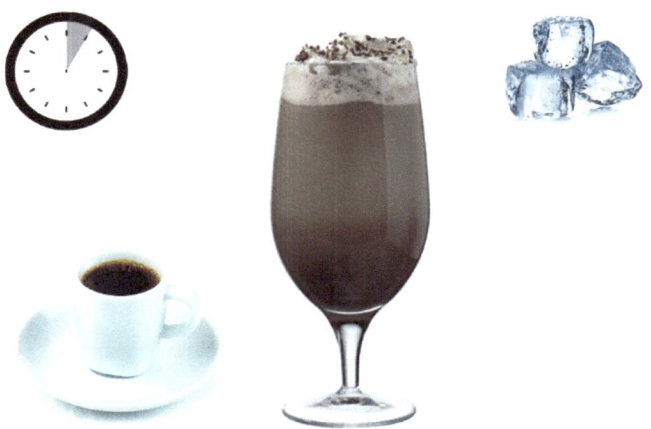

Yes, exactly you read that right. A chocolate smoothie that is healthy. It is especially helpful to make this smoothie when you have sweets craving. It will extinguish the thirst for sweets while at the same time give you a boost towards your weight loss goal.

*Mocha **Delish Recipe:***
- ***1 Espresso shot***
- ***2 cocoa powder teaspoons***
- ***½ cup of low-fat yogurt***
- ***3 ice cubes***

Add all of these ingredients in the following order: ice, yogurt, espresso, cocoa powder and blend at the highest speed until smooth.

# 12

# Raspberry Tropico

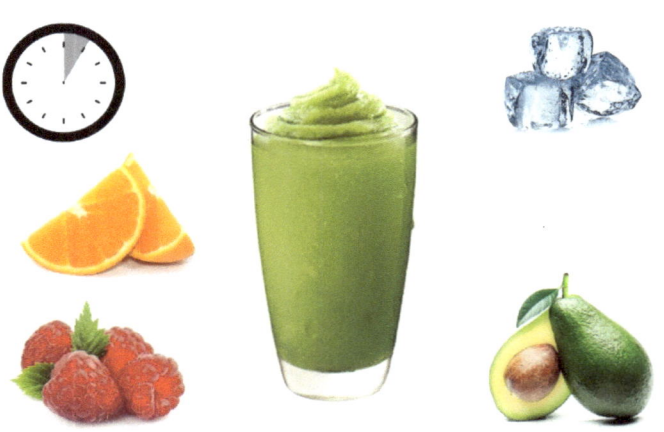

No matter how unusual this fruit combination sounds, it is one of the most delicious weight loss Smoothies that you can make in just a few minutes. The avocado will provide the perfect smoothness to this particular smoothie.

*Raspberry* **Tropico Recipe:**

- *½ cup frozen Raspberries*
- *½ cup Raspberry juice*
- *¾ cup Orange Juice*
- *1 peeled Avocado*

Just add all of the ingredients in your blender and blend to personal taste.

# 13

# Hot Tomato

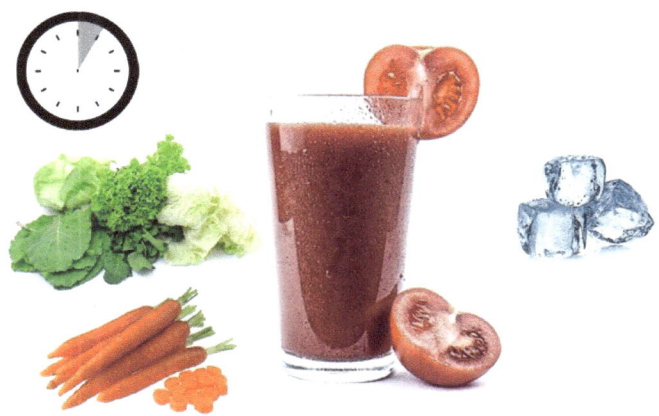

Don't be turned off because of the name of this smoothie, it's just called like that because of the Cayenne Pepper dash that is added to increase the already high level of anti-oxidants in the tomato for some extra aid in weight loss.

### Hot Tomato Smoothie Recipe:

- *¼ cup of Tomato juice*
- *9 ice cubes*
- *½ teaspoon of Cayenne pepper or any hot sauce*
- *¼ cup Apple juice*
- *¼ cup of chopped Celery*
- *½ cup of chopped Carrot*

Put everything in the blender and smoothen the mix. Enjoy

# Lime Nektar

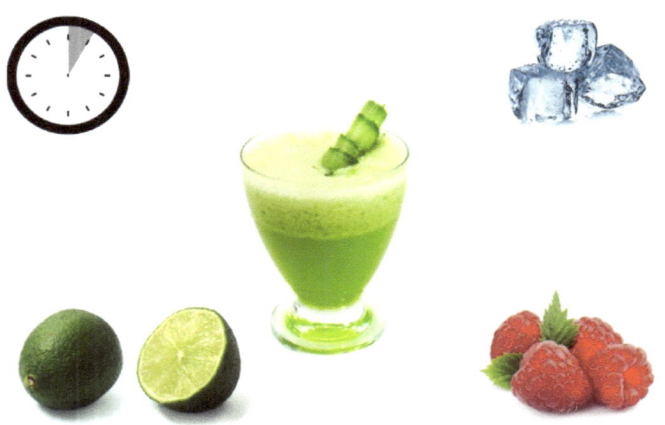

Lime as an ingredient to any smoothie will help clearing your skin and improve your digestion system drastically. Also helps with eye care and constipation problems. Don't hesitate to have a bit lime juice mixed only with warm water every morning to improve your body significantly.

*Lime* **Nektar Smoothie Recipe:**

- **½ cup sliced Lime**
- **½ cup of Lime juice**
- **½ cup fat-free soy Milk**
- **9 ice cubes**
- **½ cup raspberries**
- **And just 1 slice of Orange**

Mix everything in the blender and blend to taste.

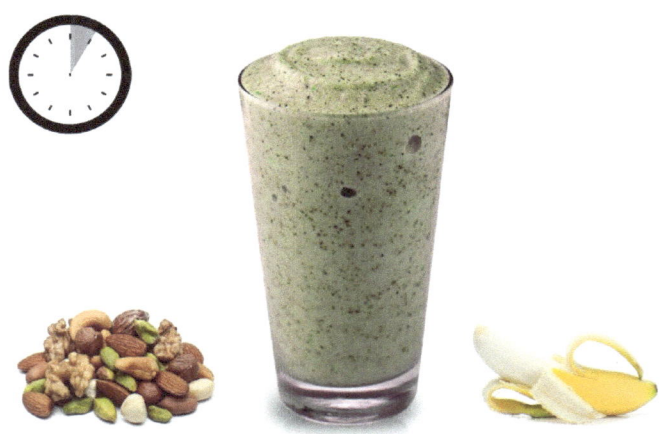

# -15-

# Nuts and Bolts

Even though the name of this smoothie sounds like something from your old garage, trust me it's one of the most delicious mixes for weight loss aid smoothies.

### Nuts and Bolts Smoothie Recipe:

- *½ cup of Pistachios and Walnuts mix*
- *1 sliced Banana*
- *½ tablespoon of Honey*
- *½ cup of non-fat yogurt*
- *½ of a teaspoon vanilla extract*

Throw everything in the Blender and Blend until smooth.

# Cantaloupe Lettuce

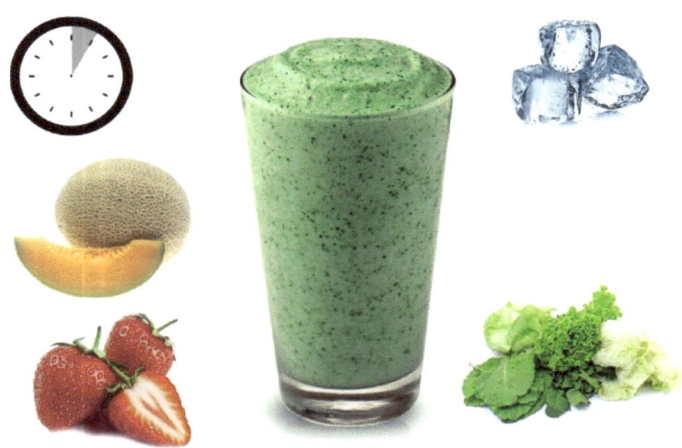

The Cantaloupe based Smoothie is rich on anti-oxidants and anti-inflammatory nutrients. Filled with organic acids, Vitamin C, Potassium this smoothie is not only good for weight loss but can also help you detoxifying and cleansing your body.

### *Cantaloupe* **Lettuce Blend Recipe:**

- *7 Lettuce leaves*
- *2 cups sliced Cantaloupe*
- *5 ice cubes*
- *1 cup of frozen strawberries*
- *½ teaspoon Cinnamon*

Place everything in the blender and blend to your own taste.

# Mix it Up

This Smoothie has more vitamins in it than I can count, and yet the proteins in it prevail for your weight loss benefit.

### *"Mix it Up" Smoothie Recipe:*
- *1 peeled Orange*
- *1 tablespoon of Honey*

- *½ of a Banana*
- *½ cup sliced Apples*
- *5 ice cubes*
- *2 Strawberries*
- *¼ cup Blueberries*

Once again mix everything in the blender and blend to your own preference.

# -18-

# Pink Spinach

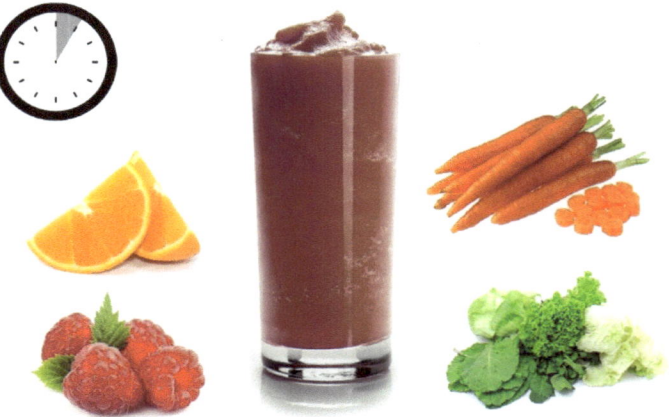

The Pink Spinach is the given name of this Smoothie personally by me. It is one of my favorite weight loss smoothie recipes that I make almost every single day, and I highly recommend it if you like to experiment with ingredients like I do.

*Pink Spinach Smoothie Recipe:*

- *1 cup of Orange Juice*
- *½ cup of fat-free Milk*
- *6-7 Spinach leaves*
- *½ teaspoon Chia seeds*
- *½ cup cold tea of your own choice*
- *1 sliced Carrot*
- *1 cup frozen Raspberries*
- *½ teaspoon Coconut oil*

Fill the ingredients in your blender and blend them all together until smooth.

# Pineapple X

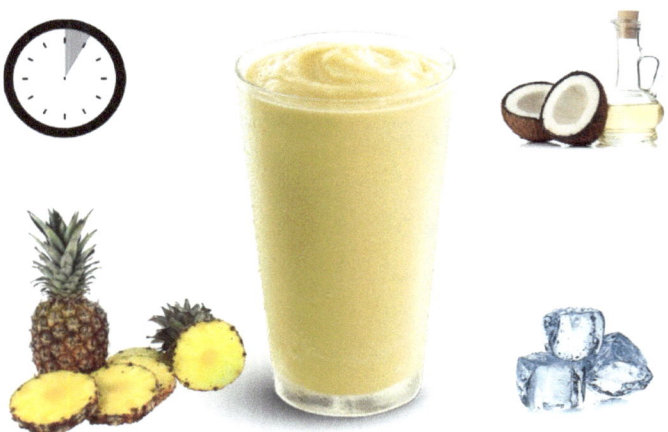

The mixture of these fruits gives one of the best looking smoothie textures, and not only that it looks good, it actually tastes even better than it looks. This easy to make smoothie will give you the daily dose of nutrients that you need.

### *Pineapple* **X Smoothie Recipe:**

- *½ Pineapple*
- *½ cup of fat-free Milk*
- *½ cup of Water*
- *3 tablespoons of non-fat yogurt*
- *5 ice cubes*
- *½ teaspoon of Coconut oil*

Blend all of the ingredients but save the Coconut oil for last, After the mix is already smooth, open the lid and add ½ teaspoon of the Coconut oil and blend for 10 seconds. Enjoy

# 20

# The Iron Kale

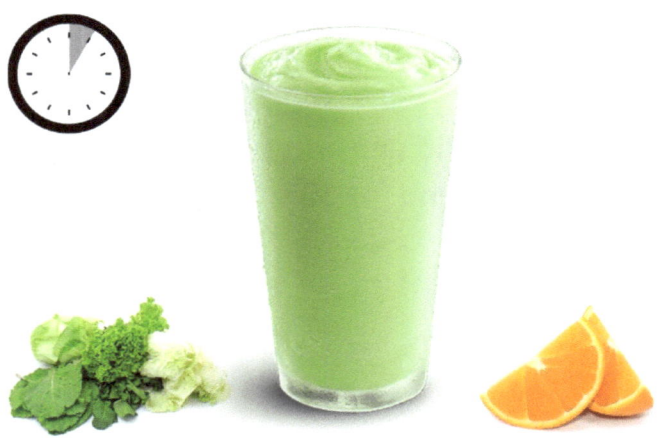

The iron and fiber vitamins packed in every sip of this smoothie will definitely make your diet easier and healthier.

### *The Iron Kale Smoothie Recipe:*
- *1 cup of raw Kale*

- *½ Orange Peeled with the seeds removed*
- *1 teaspoon Cinnamon powder*
- *1 cup of chopped Broccoli*
- *1 cup of Water*

Mix all of the ingredients together in the blender and blend until smooth.

# 21

# Tropical Veggie

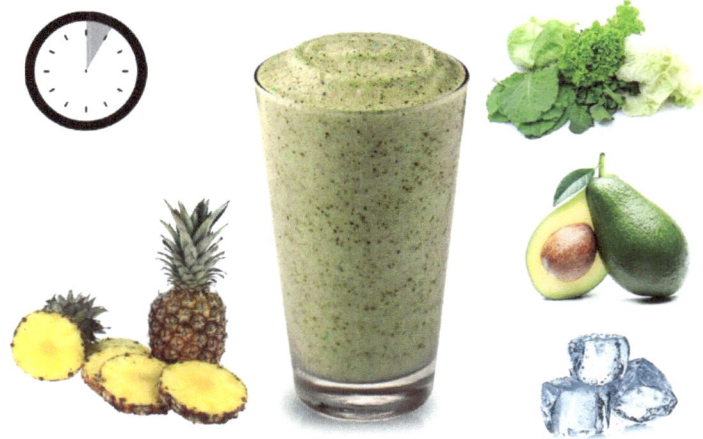

Well as they say "Last but not Least" The Tropical Veggie smoothie is packed with ingredients from two different ends of the world and I can say with confidence that this is one hell of a good weight loss combination.

Tropical Veggie Smoothie Recipe:
- 1 handful of Kale

- 1 handful of Spinach
- 1 teaspoon of Stevia sugar
- ½ cup Avocado
- ½ cup Pineapple
- ½ cup fat-free Milk
- 7 ice cubes

Place the ingredients in the blender and blend them to your own preference. Voila, you got yourself a good looking and delicious Tropical Veggie Smoothie. Enjoy.

*First of all Thank you for choosing my humble book. If you use it smart it can help you with your weight loss plan even more than you hopped for. And I know that from my personal experience.*

www.ingramcontent.com/pod-product-compliance
Lightning Source LLC
Chambersburg PA
CBHW040325010626
45792CB00024B/2146